Managing Glucose, Enhancing Life: A Step-by-Step Approach to Blood Sugar Mastery

Kevin E. Kelly

TABLE OF CONTENTS

INTRODUCTION
Understanding Blood Sugar and Its Impact on Health

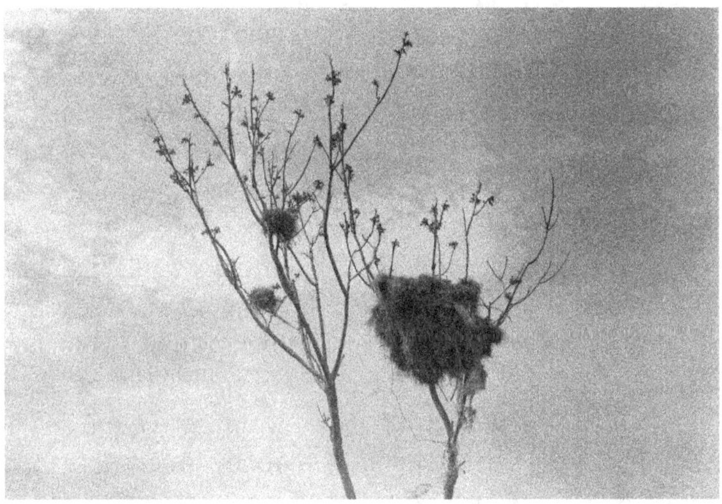

Blood sugar, also known as blood glucose, is a critical aspect of mortal health. It refers to the attention of glucose in the bloodstream, which serves as the primary source of energy for the body's cells. Proper regulation of blood sugar situations is essential for maintaining overall health and precluding colorful health conditions, especially those related to diabetes and metabolic diseases. In this comprehensive essay, we will claw into the conception of blood sugar, its part in the body, the factors impacting its situations, the impact of imbalanced blood sugar on health, and strategies to maintain healthy blood sugar situations. The Role of Blood Sugar in the Body Glucose, deduced from the food we consume, serves as the primary energy source for the body's cells. Upon digestion, carbohydrates break down into glucose, which enters the bloodstream. The pancreas, an organ located behind the stomach, plays a pivotal part in regulating blood sugar situations. When blood sugar situations rise after a mess, the pancreas releases insulin, a hormone that allows glucose to enter cells, where it's used for energy or stored for unbornuse.However, the pancreas releases glucagon, a hormone that prompts the liver to convert stored glycogen back into glucose to maintain stable blood sugar situations, If blood sugar situations drop.   Factors impacting Blood Sugar situations Several factors impact blood sugar situations, and maintaining the right balance is pivotal for overall health Diet The type and volume of carbohydrates, fats, and proteins in the diet significantly impact blood sugar situations. Simple carbohydrates, like sugars and meliorated grains, can beget rapid-fire harpoons and crashes in blood sugar situations, while complex carbohydrates, like whole grains and vegetables, lead to a more gradational and steady rise. Physical exertion Regular exercise can ameliorate insulin perceptivity, helping the body use glucose more effectively and regulate blood sugar situations more efficiently. Stress Stress hormones, similar as cortisol, can raise blood sugar situations. habitual stress may disrupt blood sugar regulation and increase the threat of developing insulin resistance. Sleep shy sleep can affect hormone regulation, leading to imbalanced blood sugar situations. Medical Conditions Certain medical conditions, like diabetes, polycystic ovary pattern(PCOS), and hormonal diseases, can impact blood sugar regulation. specifics Some specifics, similar as corticosteroids and certain antidepressants, can impact blood sugar situations. The Impact of Imbalanced Blood Sugar on Health Type 2 Diabetes Dragged ages of high blood sugar situations can lead to insulin resistance, a condition where cells come less responsive to insulin. This condition is a hallmark of type 2 diabetes. Over time, the pancreas may struggle to produce enough insulin, farther aggravating the problem. Cardiovascular Health High blood sugar situations are associated with an increased threat of cardiovascular conditions. The redundant glucose in the bloodstream can damage blood vessels, leading to atherosclerosis(the buildup of shrine) and adding the liability of heart attacks and strokes. whim-whams Damage Elevated blood sugar situations can beget whim-whams damage, known as diabetic neuropathy. This condition generally affects the bases and legs and can lead to chinking, pain, and loss of sensation. order complaint Diabetes- related order complaint, or diabetic nephropathy, is a serious complication performing from unbridled blood sugar situations. It can progress to order failure, taking dialysis or a order transplant. Vision Problems High blood sugar situations can damage the blood vessels in the eyes, leading to diabetic retinopathy, a condition that may beget vision loss or blindness. Immune System Dragged high blood sugar situations can weaken the vulnerable system, making the body more susceptible to infections. Weight Gain and rotundity Constant oscillations in blood sugar situations can spark hunger and gluttony, contributing to weight gain and rotundity. Mental Health There's a growing link between imbalanced blood sugar situations and internal health issues, similar as depression and anxiety. Strategies to Maintain Healthy Blood Sugar situations Balanced Diet Focus on a balanced diet that includes a variety of nutrient- thick foods, including whole grains, spare proteins, healthy fats, and plenitude of fruits and vegetables. Minimize the consumption of sticky potables, meliorated carbohydrates, and reused foods. Regular Exercise Engage in regular physical exertion to ameliorate insulin perceptivity and help regulate blood sugar situations. Stress operation Borrow stress-reducing ways similar as contemplation, yoga, deep breathing exercises, or pursuits to keep stress situations in check. Blood sugar is a critical aspect of mortal health, impacting colorful physiological processes and playing a central part in conditions like diabetes and metabolic diseases.

CHAPTER 1

The Importance of Blood Sugar Regulation

Blood sugar regulation is a vital physiological process that maintains glucose situations within a narrow range in the bloodstream. Glucose, the primary source of energy for the body, is attained from the food we consume. Proper blood sugar regulation is pivotal for overall health and well- being as it impacts colorful organ systems, metabolism, and plays a significant part in precluding habitual conditions. In this composition, we will explore the significance of blood sugar regulation, its mechanisms, and the consequences of its dysregulation.   The Physiology of Blood Sugar Regulation   Blood sugar regulation is an intricate process controlled by several hormones and organs in the body. The pancreas, a crucial organ, releases hormones similar as insulin and glucagon in response to changing blood glucose situations. When blood sugar situations rise after a mess, the pancreas releases insulin, which allows cells to absorb glucose, converting it into energy or storing it as glycogen in the liver and muscles. On the other hand, when blood sugar situations drop between refections or during physical exertion, the pancreas releases glucagon, which triggers the breakdown of glycogen into glucose to maintain acceptable glucose situations. Balancing Blood Sugar for Optimal Health   Maintaining stable blood sugar situations throughout the day is essential for colorful reasons   Energy situations Balanced blood sugar situations insure a steady force of glucose to cells, furnishing sustained energy and precluding oscillations that lead to fatigue and reduced productivity. Brain Function The brain is largely dependent on glucose for energy. Proper blood sugar regulation supports cognitive function, attention, and mood stability. Weight Management Stable blood sugar situations reduce the liability of gorging and jone for sticky, high- calorie foods, contributing to effective weight operation. Cardiovascular Health Chronic high blood sugar situations can damage blood vessels and increase the threat of heart complaint, stroke, and other cardiovascular issues. Diabetes Prevention Proper blood sugar regulation is vital in precluding type 2 diabetes, a condition characterized by insulin resistance and high blood sugar situations. Consequences of Blood Sugar Imbalances Hypoglycemia Low blood sugar(hypoglycemia) can beget dizziness, confusion, insecurity, and, in severe cases, loss of knowledge. Diabetics taking insulin or other glucose- lowering specifics are particularly susceptible to hypoglycemic occurrences. Hyperglycemia High blood sugar(hyperglycemia) over extended ages can lead to complications similar as diabetic ketoacidosis(DKA) in type 1 diabetes and hyperosmolar hyperglycemic state(HHS) in type 2 diabetes. These conditions can be life-hanging if not instantly treated. Insulin Resistance Dragged high blood sugar situations can lead to insulin resistance, where cells come less responsive to insulin's conduct. This condition is a precursor to class 2 diabetes and is associated with rotundity and metabolic pattern. Diabetes Mellitus undressed or inadequately managed blood sugar imbalances can lead to the development of diabetes mellitus, a habitual condition that affects millions of people worldwide and requires lifelong operation. life Factors Affecting Blood Sugar Regulation Diet Consuming a balanced diet with a focus on whole foods, complex carbohydrates, fiber, and spare proteins can help maintain stable blood sugar situations. Physical exertion Regular exercise enhances insulin perceptivity, abetting in better blood sugar control and reducing the threat of insulin resistance. Stress operation habitual stress can elevate blood sugar situations through the release of stress hormones. enforcing stress- reducing practices, similar as contemplation and awareness, can appreciatively impact blood sugar regulation. Sleep shy sleep can disrupt hormonal balance, leading to blood sugar oscillations and insulin resistance. Alcohol and Smoking inordinate alcohol consumption and smoking can negatively affect blood sugar regulation and increase the threat of metabolic diseases. Blood Sugar Regulation and Chronic conditions Type 2 Diabetes Type 2 diabetes is a current metabolic complaint characterized by insulin resistance and high blood sugar situations. Proper blood sugar regulation is pivotal for precluding and managing this condition. rotundity Imbalances in blood sugar can contribute to weight gain and rotundity. rotundity, in turn, exacerbates insulin resistance and increases the threat of developing type 2 diabetes. Cardiovascular conditions High blood sugar situations can damage blood vessels, leading to atherosclerosis and an increased threat of heart attacks and strokes. Cognitive Decline unbridled blood sugar situations have been linked to an increased threat of cognitive decline and neurodegenerative conditions like Alzheimer's.   Medical Interventions for Blood Sugar Regulatlion Insulin remedy individualities with type 1 diabetes or advanced type 2 diabetes may bear insulin   remedy to maintain proper blood sugar situations.   Oral specifics colorful oral specifics can help ameliorate blood sugar regulation by enhancing insulin perceptivity or reducing glucose product in the liver.   life variations espousing a healthy life with a focus on balanced nutrition, regular exercise, stress operation, and acceptable sleep can significantly impact blood sugar regulation.   Blood sugar regulation is a abecedarian physiological process that plays a   vital part in maintaining overall health and   precluding habitual   conditions. Proper blood sugar control is essential for energy situations, brain function, weight operation, and cardiovascular health.   The consequences of blood sugar imbalances can be severe, leading to conditions similar as diabetes, insulin resistance, and cardiovascular   conditions. By making conscious life choices, individualities can laboriously support their blood sugar regulation and   insure a healthier and   further fulfilling life. Regular medical check- ups, early discovery, and applicable interventions are pivotal for those at threat of blood sugar dysregulation or diabetes

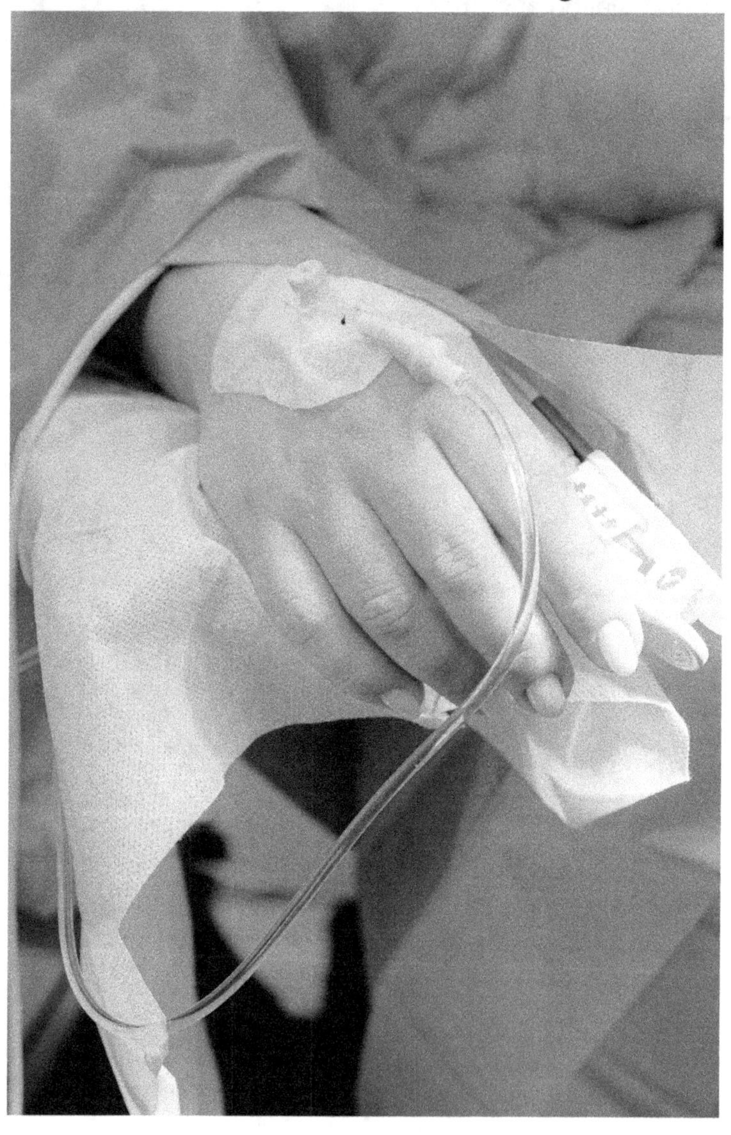

Blood sugar, or blood glucose, plays a pivotal part in maintaining the body's energy situations and overall health. still, when the balance of blood sugar is disintegrated, it can lead to colorful health issues and complications, similar as diabetes, hypoglycemia, and metabolic pattern. Understanding the common causes of blood sugar imbalance is essential for forestallment, operation, and overall well- being. In this composition, we will explore the crucial factors that contribute to blood sugar oscillations and how they can be addressed. Diet and Nutrition One of the most significant factors affecting blood sugar situations is the type and volume of food we consume. Diets high in refined carbohydrates, sugars, and reused foods can beget rapid-fire harpoons in blood glucose situations. When we eat these foods, the body releases insulin to help regulate the redundant glucose, leading to a sharp drop in blood sugar situations subsequently, which can spark hunger and Jones for further sticky foods, immortalizing the cycle. Balancing blood sugar involves choosing nutrient- thick, whole foods that are low in glycemic indicator, similar as vegetables, whole grains, spare proteins, and healthy fats. Eating lower, more frequent refections throughout the day can also help stabilize blood sugar situations. Physical exertion and Exercise Regular physical exertion and exercise are essential for maintaining healthy blood sugar situations. Exercise enhances insulin perceptivity, allowing cells to more absorb glucose for energy, which helps help blood sugar harpoons. Again, a sedentary life can contribute to insulin resistance, making it more grueling for the body to regulate blood sugar effectively. Engaging in a combination of cardiovascular exercises and strength training can be particularly salutary for blood sugar control, as it aids in weight operation and improves overall insulin perceptivity. Stress and Emotional Well-being Stress can have a profound impact on blood sugar situations due to the release of stress hormones, similar as cortisol and adrenaline. In stressful situations, the body prepares for a fight- or- flight response, leading to the release of glucose into the bloodstream for immediate energy. still, in habitual stress situations, this can disrupt the body's capability to regulate blood sugar duly. Engaging in stress- reducing conditioning like contemplation, yoga, awareness, and spending time in nature can help manage stress situations and promote emotional well- being, contributing to better blood sugar control. Sleep Patterns shy or poor- quality sleep can also affect blood sugar regulation. Sleep plays a vital part in maintaining hormonal balance, including insulin product and perceptivity. Lack of sleep can lead to insulin resistance, making it more grueling for cells to use glucose effectively. Establishing a harmonious sleep schedule, creating a comforting bedtime routine, and icing an acceptable quantum of sleep(generally 7- 9 hours for grown-ups) are essential way in promoting healthy blood sugar situations. specifics and Medical Conditions Certain specifics, similar as corticosteroids, diuretics, and beta- blockers, can intrude   with   blood   sugar   regulation,   leading toimbalances.However, it can also impact blood sugar situations, If you have a medical condition like diabetes or polycystic ovary pattern(PCOS). It's pivotal to work nearly with healthcare professionals to cover and manage blood sugar situations if you're on specifics or have an beginning medical condition. Hormonal Changes Hormonal oscillations can affect blood sugar situations, particularly in women. During the menstrual cycle, for illustration, hormones like estrogen and progesterone can impact insulin perceptivity and glucose metabolism, leading to temporary changes in blood sugar situations. Genetics and Family History Genetics can impact how our bodies handle glucose and insulin, making some individualities more predisposed to blood sugar imbalances and diabetes. A family history of diabetes or affiliated conditions can increase the threat of developing blood sugar problems. Blood sugar imbalance can have significant counteraccusations for our overall health and well-being. By understanding the common causes of blood sugar oscillations, we can take visionary way to maintain healthy blood sugar situations through life variations, similar as espousing a balanced diet, engaging in regular exercise, managing stress, prioritizing sleep, and working with healthcare professionals to address any medical conditions or specifics that may be contributing to the issue. Taking control of our blood sugar situations empowers us to live a healthier and further vibrant life.

CHAPTER 2
Blood Glucose Testing Methods

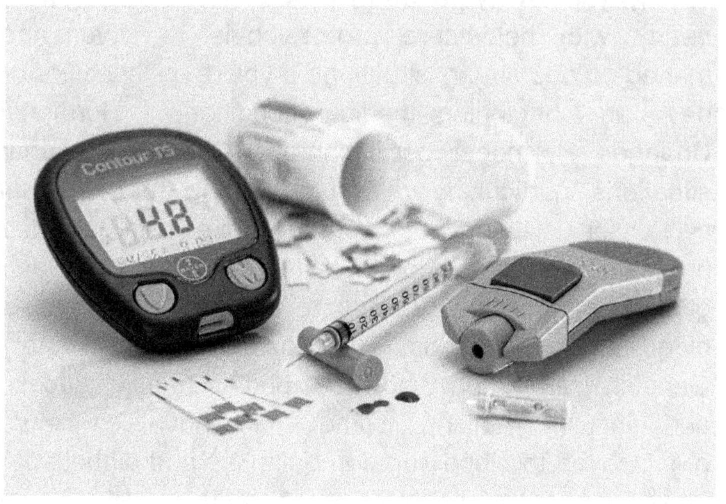

Blood glucose testing is a crucial aspect of managing diabetes and understanding overall health. It involves measuring the concentration of glucose in the bloodstream to determine a person's blood sugar level. Accurate blood glucose testing is essential for individuals with diabetes to adjust their insulin doses, monitor the effectiveness of their treatment plan, and prevent potential complications. This article aims to provide a comprehensive overview of various blood glucose testing methods, from traditional fingerstick tests to continuous glucose monitoring (CGM) systems, exploring their principles, procedures, and benefits.

Traditional Fingerstick Tests :

The traditional fingerstick method, also known as self-monitoring blood glucose (SMBG), is one of the most common ways to measure blood glucose levels. It involves pricking the fingertip with a lancet to draw a small drop of blood. This drop of blood is then placed onto a test strip that contains enzymes to react with glucose. The glucose meter reads the reaction and displays the blood glucose level on its screen within seconds.

Portable and user-friendly: SMBG devices are compact and easy to use, making them convenient for daily testing.

Quick results: Users can obtain their blood glucose levels within a few seconds.

Affordability: SMBG devices are relatively inexpensive compared to other testing methods.

Invasive: Frequent fingerstick testing can cause discomfort and lead to calluses or sore fingertips.

Limited data: Results only provide a snapshot of glucose levels at specific moments, missing patterns or trends over time.CGM systems are advanced tools that provide real-time data on glucose levels. They consist of three **main components:** a small glucose sensor inserted under the skin, a transmitter to send data wirelessly, and a receiver or smartphone app to display glucose readings.

Sensor insertion: The sensor is usually placed on the abdomen or the back of the arm. It measures glucose levels in the interstitial fluid, which correlates well with blood glucose levels.

Data transmission: The sensor continuously sends glucose data to the receiver or app at regular intervals, typically every 1 to 5 minutes.

Data display: Users can view their current glucose levels, trend lines, and alarms for hypo- or hyperglycemic events on the receiver or app.

Real-time monitoring: CGM provides a continuous stream of glucose data, allowing users to detect fluctuations and respond promptly.

Trends and patterns: CGM data can reveal glucose trends over time, helping users identify patterns and adjust their treatment plans accordingly.

Alerts and alarms: CGM systems can alert users to low or high glucose levels, enhancing safety and reducing the risk of severe hypoglycemia or hyperglycemia.

CGM systems can be more expensive than traditional SMBG methods.

Calibration: CGM sensors require periodic calibration with SMBG readings to ensure accuracy.

Flash Glucose Monitoring (FGM) Systems :

FGM systems are similar to CGM but do not provide continuous real-time data. Instead, users need to scan the sensor with a reader or smartphone app to obtain their glucose reading.

Sensor insertion: The FGM sensor is placed on the back of the upper arm and remains there for a specific period, usually up to 14 days.

Scanning: Users perform a scan over the sensor using the reader or app to receive the glucose reading and view historical data.

Convenient: Scanning is less invasive and can be done through clothing, making FGM more discreet.

Historical data: FGM systems store glucose data, allowing users to review trends over the sensor's wear period.

Delayed data: Users must actively scan the sensor to obtain glucose readings, which may result in delayed data compared to CGM.

Blood glucose testing methods play a vidiabetes effectively. Traditional fingerstick tests provide instant results but lack continuous monitoring capabilities. In contrast, CGM and FGM systems offer real-time and historical glucose data, empowering individuals with diabetes to make informed decisions about their lifestyle, medication, and insulin dosing.

For those who prefer immediate results and do not require continuous tracking, traditional SMBG may suffice. On the other hand, CGM and FGM systems are beneficial for those who want to gain deeper insights into their glucose patterns and enhance their diabetes management.

Ultimately, the choice of blood glucose testing method depends on individual needs, preferences, and financial considerations. Regular and accurate monitoring, regardless of the method chosen, is crucial for achieving optimal glucose control and preventing diabetes-related complications.

Interpreting Blood Glucose Readings

Blood glucose readings play a pivotal part in the operation of diabetes, a habitual condition characterized by the body's incapability to regulate blood sugar effectively. Understanding these readings is essential for individualities with diabetes and their healthcare providers to make informed opinions about treatment and life adaptations. This companion aims to clarify the process of interpreting blood glucose readings and empower individualities to take charge of their health.   Blood Glucose situations and Targets Blood glucose   situations are measured in milligrams per deciliter(mg/ dL) or millimoles per liter(mmol/ L). For utmost people without diabetes, a healthy fasting blood glucose   position ranges from 70- 99 mg/ dL(3.9-5.5 mmol/ L). Postprandial(after- mess) glucose situations should   immaculately stay below 140 mg/ dL(7.8 mmol/ L) two hours after eating. still, the target situations may vary depending on individual factors similar as age, diabetes type, and overall health. tone- Monitoring Blood Glucose(SMBG) individualities with diabetes   frequently perform   tone- covering blood glucose(SMBG) using a glucometer. SMBG helps track blood glucose situations throughout the day, furnishing precious perceptivity into how diet, physical exertion, drug, and stress impact blood sugar. nonstop Glucose

Monitoring(CGM) CGM is another precious tool for diabetes operation. A small detector fitted under the skin measures interstitial glucose situations continuously and displays real- time data on a receiver or smartphone. CGM provides a more comprehensive view of glucose trends, helping identify patterns and implicit issues. Patterns and Trends Interpreting blood glucose readings involves relating patterns and trends over time. High and low blood sugar occurrences should be anatomized to determine implicit triggers. constantly elevated situations(hyperglycemia) or frequent low blood sugar(hypoglycemia) may indicate the need for treatment adaptations. A1C situations The A1C test reflects average blood glucose situations over the history 2- 3 months. Expressed as a chance, an A1C target of lower than 7 is generally recommended for utmost individualities with diabetes. Lowering A1C reduces the threat of long- term complications but should be balanced with the threat of hypoglycemia. Hypoglycemia Hypoglycemia occurs when blood glucose situations drop below normal(generally below 70 mg/ dL or3.9 mmol/ L). Common symptoms include insecurity, sweating, dizziness, and confusion. It's essential to treat hypoglycemia instantly with fast- acting carbohydrates like glucose tablets or juice. Hyperglycemia Hyperglycemia is characterized by constantly high blood glucose situations. Symptoms may include increased thirst, frequent urination, fatigue, and blurred vision. unbridled hyperglycemia can lead to diabetic ketoacidosis(DKA) in type 1 diabetes or hyperosmolar hyperglycemic state(HHS) in type 2 diabetes, both of which are medical extremities. Glycemic Variability Glycemic variability refers to oscillations in blood glucose situations throughout the day. Reducing glycemic variability is important for diabetes operation as it can help help complications and promote overall well- being. Time in Range(TIR) Time in Range represents the chance of time an individual spends within a target blood glucose range, frequently set between 70- 180 mg/ dL(3.9- 10 mmol/ L). A advanced TIR is associated with better diabetes issues. Consulting Healthcare Providers Interpreting blood glucose readings isn't always straightforward, especially for those recently diagnosed with diabetes. Healthcare providers, including endocrinologists, pukka diabetes preceptors, and dietitians, play a pivotal part in guiding individualities through this process. Regular check- ups and open communication with healthcare providers are essential for effective diabetes operation. In conclusion, interpreting blood glucose readings is abecedarian to diabetes operation. It enables individualities to make informed opinions about their life, diet, and drug, eventually leading to better control of blood sugar situations and bettered overall health. By understanding these readings, individualities with diabetes can take charge of their condition and work toward a better quality of life.

CHAPTER 3

The Fundamentals of a Blood Sugar-Friendly Diet

In recent times, the frequence of diabetes and blood sugar- related diseases has surged to intimidating situations worldwide. A significant contributing factor is the ultramodern diet, which is frequently high in refined sugars, reused carbohydrates, and unhealthy fats. To promote optimal health and help blood sugar oscillations, espousing a blood sugar-friendly diet is essential. This salutary approach emphasizes whole, nutrient- thick foods and precisely considers the timing and composition of refections. In this composition, we will explore the fundamentals of a blood sugar-friendly diet and its implicit benefits in managing blood sugar situations.   Understanding Blood Sugar Regulation Before probing into the specifics of a blood sugar-friendly diet, it's essential to understand how blood sugar, or glucose, is regulated in the body. When we consume carbohydrates, they're broken down into glucose, which is also absorbed into the bloodstream. In response, the pancreas releases insulin, a hormone that helps transport glucose from the blood into the cells for energy use or storehouse. still, a diet that constantly leads to high blood sugar situations can strain the body's insulin response and contribute to insulin resistance, a precursor to diabetes. The part of Macronutrients A blood sugar-friendly diet pays particular attention to the macronutrients carbohydrates, proteins, and fats. While carbohydrates have the most significant impact on blood sugar, the other macronutrients also play vital places in overall health and blood sugar regulation. Carbohydrates Focus on consuming complex carbohydrates like whole grains, legumes, fruits, and vegetables, which are rich in fiber. Fiber slows down the immersion of glucose, precluding sharp harpoons in blood sugar situations. Proteins Including spare proteins in each mess can help stabilize blood sugar situations and promote malnutrition. Good sources of protein include flesh, fish, tofu, sap, and lentils. Fats Opt for healthy fats from sources like avocados, nuts, seeds, and olive oil painting. These fats support heart health and can help decelerate the immersion of glucose, precluding rapid-fire blood sugar oscillations. Emphasizing Low-Glycemic Foods The glycemic indicator(GI) is a measure that ranks carbohydrates grounded on their effect on blood sugar situations. Foods with a high GI cause rapid-fire harpoons in blood sugar, while those with a low GI lead to a slower, more gradational increase. A blood sugar-friendly diet prioritizes low- GI foods to promote stable blood sugar situations. exemplifications of low- GI foods include sweet potatoes, quinoa, berries, andnon-starchy vegetables. Portion Control and mess Timing piecemeal from food choices, portion control and mess timing are critical factors of a blood sugar-friendly diet. Eating large portions, indeed of healthy foods, can lead to significant blood sugar harpoons. lower, more frequent refections can help maintain more stable blood sugar situations throughout the day. also, avoiding long gaps between refections can help gluttony and blood sugar imbalances. barring or Limiting Sugary potables and Processed Foods Sugar- candied potables, similar as tonics, fruit authorities, and energy drinks, are loaded with added sugars and snappily raise blood sugar situations. These should be avoided or limited in a blood sugar-friendly diet. also, reused foods frequently contain retired sugars, unhealthy fats, and meliorated carbohydrates, all of which can disrupt blood sugar regulation. concluding for whole, undressed foods is the stylish approach to maintain stable blood sugar situations and overall health. aware Eating and Blood Sugar Management aware eating is an essential practice in a blood sugar-friendly diet. It involves paying attention to hunger cues, eating sluggishly, and savoring each bite. By being aware of the eating process, individualities can help gluttony and better fete when they're truly quenched. The significance of Regular Physical exertion Physical exertion is a important tool in blood sugar operation. Regular exercise helps ameliorate insulin perceptivity, allowing the body to use glucose more effectively. Engaging in a combination of aerobic exercises, strength training, and inflexibility exercises can have significant benefits for blood sugar regulation. Hydration and Blood Sugar Staying doused is pivotal for overall health and blood sugar operation. Water is the stylish choice for hydration, as it doesn't impact blood sugar situations.

Avoid sticky drinks and inordinate alcohol consumption, both of which can beget blood sugar oscillations. A blood sugar-friendly diet is centered around total, nutrient- thick foods, balanced macronutrients, and aware eating practices. By fastening on low- GI foods, portion control, and regular physical exertion, individualities can help regulate their blood sugar situations and promote overall well- being. Embracing this salutary approach can be a significant step towards precluding blood sugar imbalances and reducing the threat of diabetes and affiliated health complication

Creating a Personalized Meal Plan

Creating a personalized meal plan is a powerful approach to optimize nutrition, promote overall well-being, and achieve specific health and fitness goals. A personalized meal plan takes into account an individual's unique requirements, preferences, and lifestyle to design a balanced and sustainable diet that meets their nutritional needs. This comprehensive guide outlines the key steps involved in creating a personalized meal plan.

Set Clear Goals

The first step in creating a personalized meal plan is to define clear and achievable goals. These goals could be related to weight management, athletic performance, managing specific health conditions, or simply improving overall nutrition. Understanding the objectives will serve as a foundation for designing a meal plan that aligns with the individual's desired outcomes.

Assess Current Health and Dietary Habits

Before crafting a personalized meal plan, it's essential to evaluate an individual's current health status and dietary habits. This assessment may include factors such as age, gender, weight, height, activity level, medical history, allergies, and food preferences. Gathering this information helps identify specific dietary needs and potential areas for improvement.

Calculate Caloric Needs

Determining an individual's daily caloric needs is crucial to create a well-balanced meal plan. The total daily energy expenditure (TDEE) takes into account basal metabolic rate (BMR) and activity level. Online calculators or consulting with a registered dietitian can help accurately estimate caloric needs based on individual characteristics and goals.

Identify Nutritional Requirements

After calculating caloric needs, the next step is to define the appropriate macronutrient ratios and micronutrient requirements for the individual. Macronutrients include carbohydrates, proteins, and fats, while micronutrients encompass essential vitamins and minerals. These requirements can vary depending on factors like age, gender, activity level, and specific health conditions.

Plan Balanced Meals

A balanced meal plan should incorporate a variety of foods to ensure all essential nutrients are provided. Meals should contain a mix of lean proteins, whole grains, healthy fats, fruits, vegetables, and dairy or dairy alternatives. The portion sizes and distribution of macronutrients can be adjusted to meet individual needs and preferences while maintaining overall balance.

Consider Dietary Restrictions and Allergies

Individuals may have specific dietary restrictions or allergies that must be considered when creating a personalized meal plan. For instance, some people might be lactose intolerant, have celiac disease, or follow a vegetarian or vegan lifestyle. Adapting the meal plan to accommodate these requirements is essential to ensure optimal health and adherence.

Include Regular Snacks

Incorporating snacks between meals is beneficial for maintaining stable energy levels and preventing overeating during main meals. Snacks should be nutrient-dense and aligned with the individual's dietary goals. Balanced options such as nuts, yogurt, fruit, or whole-grain crackers can be chosen as healthy snacks.

Hydration is Key

Staying adequately hydrated is often overlooked but plays a crucial role in overall health. The personalized meal plan should include recommendations for daily water intake based on individual factors like activity level, climate, and body weight.

Gradual Implementation and Adjustments

Transitioning to a personalized meal plan should be a gradual process to allow the body to adapt and minimize any potential discomfort. Regular monitoring and adjustments may be necessary as factors like weight loss or increased physical activity can influence dietary requirements.

Monitor Progress

Continuously monitoring progress is essential for the success of the personalized meal plan. Regularly evaluating changes in weight, energy levels, performance, and overall well-being will help identify the plan's effectiveness and make any necessary modifications.

Creating a personalized meal plan is a holistic process that takes into account an individual's unique needs, preferences, and objectives. By setting clear goals, assessing current health and dietary habits, calculating caloric needs, and identifying nutritional requirements, a well-balanced and sustainable meal plan can be designed. Integrating dietary restrictions, including regular snacks, staying hydrated, and making gradual adjustments further enhances the effectiveness of the plan. Regular monitoring and adjustments ensure continued progress and success in achieving health and fitness goals.

CHAPTER 4
Meal Planning and Portion Control

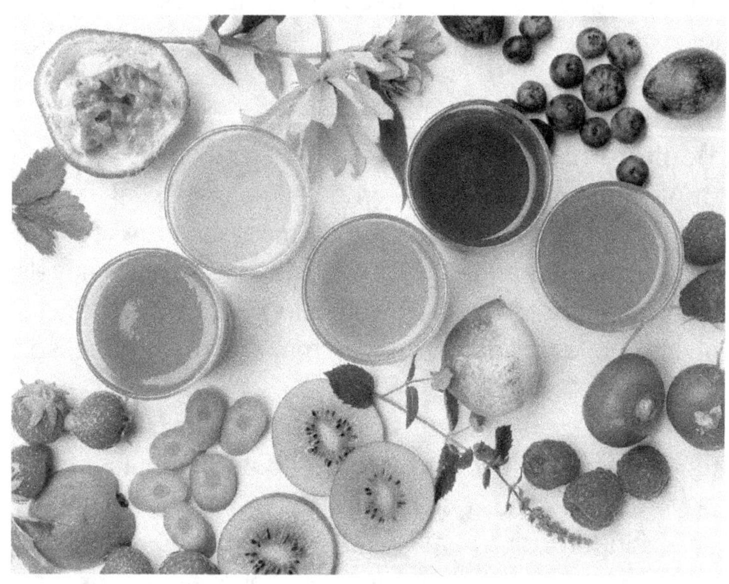

Maintaining stable blood glucose situations is vital for overall health, especially for individualities with diabetes or those at threat of developing the condition. mess planning and portion control play pivotal places in managing glucose situations effectively. by making informed choices about the types and amounts of food consumed, individualities can regulate their blood sugar situations, minimize harpoons, and reduce the threat of complications associated with glucose imbalances. this composition explores the principles of mess planning and portion control that contribute to better glucose operation. understanding glucose and its part glucose, a simple sugar, is the primary source of energy for the body's cells. it enters the bloodstream through the digestion of carbohydrates in the foods we eat. insulin, a hormone produced by the pancreas, allows glucose to enter the cells, where it's used for energy. in individualities with diabetes or insulin resistance, the body struggles to regulate glucose effectively, leading to elevated blood sugar situations. the significance of mess planning mess planning involves thoughtful consideration of the types and amounts of foods consumed throughout the day. it aims to balance carbohydrate input with the body's insulin response, promoting stable blood glucose situations. then are some essential aspects of effective mess planning for glucose operation carbohydrate mindfulness carbohydrates have the most significant impact on blood glucose situations. knowing the carbohydrate content of different foods and understanding how they affect blood sugar is pivotal. it's essential to concentrate on complex carbohydrates set up in whole grains, vegetables, and legumes, while limiting simple carbohydrates from sticky and reused foods. balanced refections a well- balanced mess should include a combination of carbohydrates, proteins, and healthy fats. proteins and fats help decelerate down the immersion of carbohydrates, precluding rapid-fire harpoons in blood glucose situations. harmonious eating schedule maintaining regular mess times can help stabilize blood glucose situations. avoid skipping refections or going for long ages without eating, as it can lead to oscillations in blood sugar. glycemic indicator(gi) mindfulness the glycemic indicator measures how snappily a carbohydrate- containing food raises blood glucose situations. foods with a low gi are preferable, as they beget slower, more gradational increases in blood sugar. the part of portion control portion control is another critical aspect of glucose operation. indeed healthy foods can negatively impact blood glucose situations if consumed in inordinate quantities. then is how portion control can help   avoid gorging consuming large portions of any food, especially high- carbohydrate particulars, can lead to dramatic harpoons in blood glucose   situations. controlling portion sizes helps manage these oscillations. read nutrition markers pay attention to serving sizes mentioned on nutrition markers. frequently, packaged foods contain multiple servings, and consuming the whole package can lead to inordinate carbohydrate input. use lower plates eating from lower plates and coliseums can produce an vision of a fuller plate, helping control portion sizes and help gluttony.   hear to hunger cues eating mindfully and feting malnutrition signals can help intemperance. conclusion effective glucose operation through mess planning and portion control is pivotal for individualities with diabetes or those aiming to maintain stable blood sugar situations. being aware of carbohydrate input, choosing balanced   refections, and understanding portion sizes are all essential   factors of successful glucose operation. also, regular physical exertion and close monitoring of blood glucose situations round these salutary strategies, enabling individualities to lead healthier lives while keeping glucose situations in check. always consult with a healthcare professional or a registered dietitian to produce a substantiated mess plan that suits individual requirements and medical conditions. by taking visionary way towards glucose operation, individualities can enhance their overall well-being and reduce the threat of diabetes- related complication.

Smart Snacking for Stable Blood Sugar

Maintaining stable blood sugar situations is essential for overall health and well- being. It's particularly pivotal for individualities with diabetes or those at threat of developing the condition. One effective way to regulate blood sugar situations is through smart snacking. By making thoughtful choices and understanding how different foods impact blood sugar, individualities can enjoy snacks that support stable glucose situations and give sustained energy throughout the day. The significance of Stable Blood Sugar situations Blood sugar, or glucose, is the primary source of energy for the body's cells. still, sharp oscillations in blood sugar situations can lead to adverse health goods, similar as fatigue, mood swings, and increased threat of developing diabetes. Stable blood sugar situations are pivotal for maintaining a harmonious force of energy and reducing the threat of habitual conditions. Choose Complex Carbohydrates When gorging, it's essential to conclude for complex carbohydrates rather of simple sugars. Complex carbs, set up in whole grains, fruits, and vegetables, take longer to digest, leading to a slower and further gradational increase in blood sugar situations. This sustained release of glucose helps help unforeseen harpoons and crashes, furnishing a more stable source of energy. Fiber is Your Friend Fiber plays a significant part in stabilizing blood sugar situations. High- fiber snacks, like nuts, seeds, and fruits, decelerate down the immersion of glucose and promote better glycemic control. also, fiber-rich snacks can help with malnutrition, precluding gluttony and supporting healthy weight operation. Include Healthy Fats Incorporating healthy fats into your snacks can also help regulate blood sugar. Fats laggardly down the digestion of food, performing in a further gradational increase in glucose situations. Avocado, nuts, seeds, and olives are excellent sources of monounsaturated and polyunsaturated fats, which contribute to heart health and blood sugar stability. Brace Carbs with Proteins When gorging, consider combining carbohydrates with proteins. Proteins can help decelerate down the immersion of glucose, reducing the impact on blood sugar situations. exemplifications of smart snack combinations include apple slices with peanut adulation, whole- grain crackers with hummus, or Greek yogurt with berries. Avoid largely Reused Snacks largely reused snacks frequently contain refined sugars, unhealthy fats, and warrant essential nutrients. These types of snacks can beget rapid-fire harpoons in blood sugar situations, followed by a crash, leaving you feeling tired and empty. conclude for whole, nutrient- thick foods as snacks rather. Portion Control Indeed healthy snacks can impact blood sugar situations if consumed in inordinate quantities. Pay attention to portion sizes, and avoid mindlessly eating directly from large bags or holders. Pre-portioning snacks can help you stick to appropriate serving sizes and help intemperance. aware Eating rehearsing aware eating can appreciatively impact blood sugar regulation. Take time to savor your snacks, chew sluggishly, and be apprehensive of hunger cues and malnutrition signals. Eating mindfully can help gluttony and help you make better snack choices. Hydration Matters Staying doused is vital for overall health and can impact blood sugar situations as well. Drinking plenitude of water throughout the day can help help inordinate thirst and potentially reduce the threat of consuming sticky potables or snacks out of thirst. Examiner and Acclimate Each person's response to different foods may vary, so it's essential to cover your blood sugar situations after gorging and make adaptations as necessary. Keeping a food journal can help identify which snacks work stylish for you and which bones may lead to oscillations in blood sugar. smart snacking is a precious tool for maintaining stable blood sugar situations and supporting overall health. By choosing nutrient- thick, whole foods, and paying attention to portion sizes, individualities can enjoy snacks that give sustained energy and promote optimal blood sugar regulation. Incorporating these smart snacking habits into your diurnal routine can lead to bettered well- being and reduced threat of habitual health conditions associated with unstable blood sugar situations.

CHAPTER 5
Exercise and Physical Activity for Blood Sugar Control

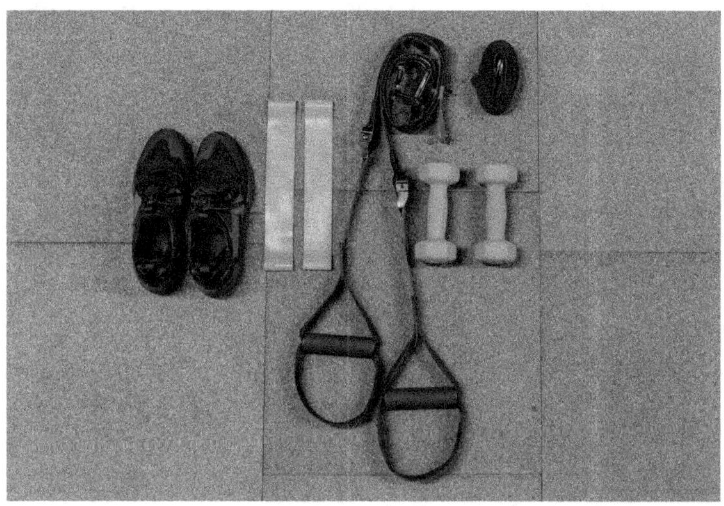

Physical Exertion and exercise play a pivotal part in managing blood sugar situations and precluding diabetes- related complications. Diabetes, a habitual metabolic complaint characterized by high blood sugar situations, affects millions of people worldwide. Type 2 diabetes, the most current form, is frequently associated with life factors, including sedentary geste and poor salutary habits. Incorporating regular exercise and physical exertion into bone's diurnal routine can have a profound impact on blood sugar control and overall health. The Link Between Exercise and Blood Sugar When we engage in physical exertion, our muscles bear energy in the form of glucose. To meet this demand, the body increases insulin perceptivity, allowing glucose to enter the cells more efficiently. This process helps to lower blood sugar situations. also, exercise can lead to weight loss or weight conservation, which is especially salutary for people with type 2 diabetes, as redundant weight can contribute to insulin resistance.   Types of Exercise for Blood Sugar Control colorful types of exercise can be effective in managing blood sugar situations. Aerobic exercises, similar as walking, jogging, swimming, and cycling, are particularly helpful as they increase heart rate and respiratory exertion, leading to bettered glucose application. Strength training exercises, involving resistance training with weights or bodyweight exercises, also have a positive impact. Muscle- strengthening exercises enhance insulin perceptivity, promoting better blood sugar regulation.   Timing and Duration of Exercise The timing and duration of exercise can impact its goods on blood sugar control. numerous studies suggest that moderate- intensity aerobic exercise for at least 150 twinkles per week, spread across several days, is salutary. It's essential to find a routine that suits an existent's preferences and life. For some, shorter, more violent exercises might be preferable, while others may enjoy longer, moderate exercises. Chronicity is crucial, and thickness in exercise habits can lead to lasting benefits. Preventives and Considerations   Before starting an exercise authority, individualities with diabetes should consult their healthcare provider. Some preventives and considerations include   Blood Sugar Monitoring Regularly covering blood sugar situations ahead, during, and after exercise helps understand how physical exertion affects the body. This information allows for better adaptations to insulin boluses or carbohydrate input. Hydration Staying well-doused is essential during exercise, as dehumidification can affect blood sugar situations. Drinking water before, during, and after exercise is pivotal. Hypoglycemia Physical exertion can occasionally lead to hypoglycemia(low blood sugar). It's important to be prepared by carrying presto- acting carbohydrates like glucose tablets or energy gels to treat low blood sugar if demanded. Foot Care People with diabetes should pay close attention to bottom care, icing proper footwear and regular bottom examinations to help complications. Personalized Approach Different individualities may respond else to exercise. It's essential to knitter the exercise routine to individual preferences, fitness position, and medical history. Combining Exercise with Diet While exercise alone can significantly impact blood sugar control, combining it with a healthy diet can amplify the benefits. A balanced diet that includes whole grains, spare proteins, fruits, vegetables, and healthy fats complements physical exertion by furnishing essential nutrients and maintaining steady blood sugar situations. Long- Term Benefits Regular exercise and physical exertion not only help manage blood sugar situations but also offer a range of long- term benefits for individualities with diabetes. These include

Cardiovascular Health Exercise improves heart health by reducing the threat of cardiovascular conditions, which are frequently associated with diabetes. Weight Management Maintaining a healthy weight reduces insulin resistance and improves blood sugar regulation. Stress Reduction Physical exertion helps reduce stress, which can have positive goods on blood sugar situations.   Overall Well- being Regular exercise can boost energy situations, ameliorate mood, and enhance overall quality of life.   Exercise and physical exertion are important tools in blood sugar control for people with diabetes. The positive impact of exercise on insulin perceptivity, glucose application, and weight operation can not be exaggerated. With applicable preventives and substantiated approaches, individualities can integrate exercise into their diurnal routines, leading to better blood sugar control and bettered overall health.

Developing a Sustainable Workout Routine

Creating a sustainable drill routine is essential for long- term health, fitness, and overall well- being. A well- structured and balanced approach to exercise not only helps in achieving fitness pretensions but also ensures thickness, precluding collapse and injuries. In this companion, we will explore the crucial principles and way to develop a sustainable drill routine that you can maintain for the long haul.   Set Clear pretensions Before embarking on any fitness trip, it's vital to establish clear and realistic pretensions. Whether it's perfecting cardiovascular health, structure muscle, losing weight, or enhancing inflexibility, understanding your objects will shape your drill routine consequently. Set both short- term and long- term pretensions to keep yourself motivated throughout the trip. Assess Your Fitness position Knowing your current fitness position is pivotal for designing a routine that suits your capabilities. Conduct a fitness assessment to estimate your strength, inflexibility, abidance, and overall health. This evaluation will help you identify your strengths and sins, enabling you to conform the drill plan to suit your individual requirements. Incorporate Variety Variety is the spice of life, and it also applies to fitness routines. Engaging in different types of exercises not only prevents humdrum but also targets colorful muscle groups, promoting overall fitness. Consider including a blend of cardiovascular exercises, strength training, inflexibility exercises, and conditioning that you authentically enjoy to keep your interest piqued. launch Slow and Progress Gradationally One of the most common miscalculations in drill routines is trying to do too much too soon. Starting slow and gradationally adding the intensity and duration of your exercises is essential for precluding injuries and collapse. hear to your body and be patient with the progress. Incremental advancements over time will yield better and further sustainable results. Schedule Regular Rest Days Rest and recovery are just as pivotal as exercise itself. Your body needs time to repair and rebuild muscle apkins after emphatic exercises. Incorporate regular rest days into your routine to help overtraining and reduce the threat of injury. Rest also helps maintain provocation and prevents drill fatigue. produce a Balanced Routine A sustainable drill routine should be well- balanced, targeting different aspects of fitness. Aim to include cardiovascular exercises to ameliorate abidance, strength training for muscle development, and inflexibility exercises to enhance mobility. Consider incorporating conditioning that support internal well-being, similar as yoga or contemplation, to produce a holistic approach to fitness. hear to Your Body Your body is your stylish companion in any fitness trip. Pay attention to how you feel during and afterworkouts.However, it's essential to address the issue rather than pushing through, If you witness pain or discomfort. Seek professional advice when demanded and modify your routine consequently. Being in tune with your body will help you make informed opinions for a sustainable drill plan. Make it pleasurable Enjoyment is the key tosustainability.However, you're less likely to stick to your routine in the long run, If you find your exercises tedious or unwelcome. Find conditioning you authentically enjoy, whether it's dancing, hiking, swimming, or playing asport.However, staying harmonious will come a natural part of your life, If you look forward to your exercises. Set a Realistic Schedule Time constraints can frequently hamper drill thickness. Be realistic about your schedule and commitments when designing your routine. Set away devoted time for exercise, indeed if it's just a many twinkles a day. thickness is more important than duration, so indeed short exercises can yield positive results if done regularly.   Track Your Progress Monitoring your progress is essential for staying motivated and making adaptations as demanded. Keep a drill journal or use fitness apps to record your exercises, duration, and intensity. Take periodic measures and track changes in your fitness position. Celebrate your achievements and use lapses as learning openings to upgrade your routine further. Conclusion   Developing a sustainable drill routine is a trip that requires fidelity, tolerance, and tone-mindfulness. By setting clear pretensions, being aware of your body, and incorporating variety and balance, you can produce a drill plan that fits your individual requirements and preferences. Flash back that sustainability isn't just about short- term earnings but about establishing a life that supports your well- being for times to come. Stay married, stay motivated, and enjoy the numerous benefits of a harmonious and sustainable drill routine.

CHAPTER 6

The Mind-Body Connection

The mind-body connection is a complex and fascinating phenomenon that highlights the intricate relationship between our mental and physical states. It refers to the powerful interplay between our thoughts, emotions, beliefs, and attitudes with our physiological responses and overall health. Understanding how the mind and body influence each other can have profound implications for our well-being and the management of various health conditions.

At the core of the mind-body connection is the central nervous system, comprising the brain and spinal cord, which acts as the communication hub between the mind and the body. The brain plays a pivotal role in processing information, interpreting emotions, and generating thoughts. When we experience stress, fear, or joy, the brain releases neurotransmitters and hormones that signal the body to respond accordingly.

One significant pathway in the mind-body connection is the hypothalamic-pituitary-adrenal (HPA) axis. When the brain perceives a threat or stressor, the hypothalamus signals the pituitary gland to release adrenocorticotropic hormone (ACTH), which then prompts the adrenal glands to produce stress hormones like cortisol. These stress hormones prepare the body for a "fight or flight" response, raising heart rate, increasing blood pressure, and mobilizing energy stores.

The immune system is also influenced by the mind-body connection. Psychological stress can affect immune function, making individuals more susceptible to infections and illnesses. Chronic stress may lead to inflammation and immune system dysregulation, contributing to the development of autoimmune disorders and other health problems.

Moreover, the mind can influence the body through the placebo and nocebo effects. When individuals believe they are receiving a treatment, even if it's a sugar pill with no therapeutic properties, their mind can trigger biochemical changes that lead to real physiological improvements. On the contrary, the nocebo effect occurs when negative expectations or beliefs about a treatment or situation result in adverse outcomes.

Emotions play a significant role in the mind-body connection. Positive emotions like happiness and contentment have been linked to better overall health, improved cardiovascular function, and enhanced immune response. Conversely, chronic negative emotions like anger, anxiety, and depression can have detrimental effects on the body, increasing the risk of heart disease, metabolic disorders, and other health issues.

The mind-body connection can also influence chronic pain conditions. Pain perception involves complex interactions between the brain, spinal cord, and nerves. Emotional factors, such as fear and stress, can amplify pain perception, leading to a cycle of heightened pain experiences. Mind-body practices like meditation, mindfulness, and cognitive-behavioral therapy have shown promising results in managing chronic pain by addressing the psychological aspects of pain.

Additionally, the mind-body connection extends to the gastrointestinal system, often referred to as the "second brain" due to its extensive neural network. Stress and emotions can impact gut function, contributing to digestive disorders like irritable bowel syndrome (IBS). Conversely, imbalances in the gut microbiome can influence mental health conditions like anxiety and depression, underscoring the bidirectional nature of the mind-body connection.

Several practices can harness the power of the mind-body connection for better health and well-being. Mindfulness and meditation techniques promote present-moment awareness, reduce stress, and enhance emotional regulation. Exercise not only benefits the body physically but also improves mood and cognitive function, fostering a positive mind-body loop.

Mind-body connection is a complex and dynamic interaction between our mental and physical states. The brain, nervous system, hormones, and emotions all play pivotal roles in this intricate relationship. Understanding and utilizing the mind-body connection can have transformative effects on our overall health and quality of life, highlighting the profound impact that our thoughts and emotions can have on our well-being. By nurturing a positive and balanced mind-body connection through practices like mindfulness, meditation, and exercise, we can pave the way for a healthier and more fulfilling life.

Mindfulness and Meditation for Blood Sugar Management

Managing blood sugar situations is pivotal for individualities with diabetes or those at threat of developing the condition. While diet and exercise play a significant part in blood sugar operation, the objectification of awareness and contemplation into bone's diurnal routine can offer profound benefits. awareness and contemplation promote tone-mindfulness, stress reduction, and emotlonal balance, all of which appreciatively impact blood sugar regulation. In this composition, we will explore how to integrate awareness and contemplation practices into your life to support blood sugar operation. Understanding awareness and Contemplation awareness is the practice of being completely present in the moment, observing studies, passions, and sensations without judgment. Contemplation, on the other hand, involves fastening attention and barring distractions. Both practices partake common rudiments and round each other. By incorporating awareness and contemplation, you can cultivate a deeper connection with your body and feelings, leading to better blood sugar control. aware Eating aware eating involves paying close attention to the sensitive experience of eating. Take time to appreciate the flavors, textures, and aromas of your food. Bite sluggishly and savor each bite. By eating mindfully, you can avoid gluttony and make healthier food choices, eventually contributing to more blood sugar operation. Stress Reduction Stress can significantly impact blood sugar situations. When stressed, the body releases hormones like cortisol and adrenaline, which can beget blood sugar harpoons. awareness and contemplation are important tools to manage stress. Engage in diurnal awareness practices, similar as deep breathing exercises or progressive muscle relaxation, to reduce stress and its negative goods on blood sugar. Emotional Regulation Emotional paroxysms can lead to emotional eating and erratic blood sugar situations. Through awareness and contemplation, you can develop emotional regulation chops, feting and accepting feelings without letting them overwhelm you. When faced with grueling feelings, take a moment to breathe deeply, observe your passions, and allow them to pass without judgment. Regular Meditation Sessions Set away time each day for contemplation. Find a quiet space, sit comfortably, and concentrate on your breath or use guided contemplation ways. Contemplation promotes relaxation and reduces the body's stress response, contributing to better blood sugar control. awareness in Physical Conditioning Whether it's walking, yoga, or other exercises, practice awareness during physical conditioning. Pay attention to your body's movements and sensations. aware exercise can enhance your connection to your body, helping you fete signs of low or high blood sugar during or after the drill. awareness in Daily Conditioning Integrate awareness into your diurnal routine by being completely present in everyday tasks. Whether you are brushing your teeth, washing dishes, or exchanging to work, concentrate on the present moment. This habit reinforces awareness throughout the day, reducing stress and supporting better blood sugar regulation.   Mindfulness Group or Community Join a awareness or contemplation group or community. participating gests and learning from others can enhance your practice and give a support network. also, engaging with suchlike- inclined individualities fosters provocation and liability. Incorporating awareness and contemplation into your life can have a significant positive impact on blood sugar operation. By rehearsing awareness in eating, stress reduction, emotional regulation, and diurnal conditioning, you can achieve better control over your blood sugar situations. Regular contemplation sessions further enhance these benefits, fostering a deeper mind- body connection and overall well- being. Flash back that thickness is crucial, and over time, the civilization of awareness and contemplation practices can lead to lasting advancements in your health and quality of life. Always consult with your healthcare provider before making any significant changes to your diabetes operation routine.

CHAPTER 7

Understanding the Sleep-Blood Sugar Connection

Sleep and blood sugar regulation are two vital aspects of mortal health that are intricately connected. The intricate relationship between sleep and blood sugar situations plays a significant part in overall well- being and can impact colorful aspects of health, including metabolism, weight operation, and diabetes threat. In this composition, we will explore the sleep- blood sugar connection, the physiological mechanisms involved, and the counteraccusations for health.

1. The Basics of Blood Sugar Regulation Before probing into the sleep- blood sugar connection, it's essential to grasp the fundamentals of blood sugar regulation. Blood sugar, also known as blood glucose, is the primary source of energy for our body's cells. After we consume food, especially carbohydrates, our digestive system breaks down these nutrients into glucose motes that enter the bloodstream. In response to rising blood glucose   situations, the pancreas releases insulin, a hormone that enables cells to take in glucose for energy use or storehouse.

2. Sleep and Circadian measures   The mortal body operates on a 24- hour internal timepiece known as the circadian   meter. This internal   timepiece regulates multitudinous physiological processes, including the sleep- wake cycle. The circadian meter is primarily told by environmental cues, similar as light and darkness, and is coordinated by a region of the brain called the suprachiasmatic nexus.

3. Impact of Sleep on Blood Sugar situations Research has constantly shown that sleep plays a pivotal part in blood sugar regulation. Both the volume and quality of sleep can impact blood glucose situations, insulin perceptivity, and the threat of developing insulin resistance and type 2 diabetes. Then is how sleep affects blood sugar situations Sleep Duration Getting an acceptable quantum of sleep is essential for maintaining healthy blood sugar situations. Short sleep duration has been associated with elevated blood glucose situations and reduced insulin perceptivity. habitual sleep privation can lead to insulin resistance, adding the threat of type 2 diabetes over time. Sleep Quality Indeed if an existent gets the recommended quantum of sleep, poor sleep quality can still impact blood sugar regulation. Sleep disturbances, similar as frequent awakenings or sleep apnea, can disrupt the circadian meter and vitiate glucose metabolism, leading to dysregulation of blood sugar situations. Circadian dislocation Shift work, spurt pause, and irregular sleep schedules can disrupt the circadian meter, impacting the body's capability to regulate blood sugar effectively. Night shift workers, for illustration, frequently face advanced pitfalls of developing metabolic diseases due to disturbances in their sleep-wake cycles. Hormonal Imbalance Sleep plays a part in regulating colorful hormones, including insulin, cortisol, and growth hormones. Poor sleep can lead to imbalances in these hormones, which may contribute to abnormal blood sugar situations and increased diabetes threat.

4. Mechanisms Behind the Sleep- Blood Sugar Connection Sympathetic Nervous System During deep sleep, the sympathetic nervous system, which controls the body's stress response, becomes less active. Reduced SNS exertion at night allows the parasympathetic nervous system(PNS), responsible for rest and digestion, to dominate. This shift promotes glucose uptake and storehouse, helping to maintain blood sugar situations within a healthy range. Growth Hormone Release Deep sleep stages, particularly during the first half of the night, are associated with the release of growth hormone. This hormone aids in towel form and glucose metabolism, helping to regulate blood sugar situations during sleep. Cortisol situations Cortisol, frequently appertained to as the" stress hormone," follows a natural circadian pattern, with its peak generally being in the early morning. still, disintegrated sleep can lead to abnormal cortisol stashing, contributing to insulin resistance and disabled blood sugar regulation. Melatonin Melatonin, a hormone responsible for promoting sleep, also influences glucose metabolism. Studies have shown that melatonin supplementation may ameliorate insulin perceptivity, suggesting a implicit link between melatonin situations and blood sugar regulation.

5. Counteraccusations for Health Diabetes Risk constantly poor sleep patterns and sleep privation are associated with an increased threat of developing type 2 diabetes. Addressing sleep issues may be a precious approach in diabetes forestallment and operation. rotundity and Weight Management disintegrated sleep can lead to differences in hunger hormones, increased appetite, and poor food choices, contributing to weight gain and rotundity. perfecting sleep quality and duration can appreciatively impact weight operation sweats. Cardiovascular Health Sleep disturbances and poor blood sugar control are linked to an elevated threat of cardiovascular conditions, similar as hypertension and heart complaint. Prioritizing healthy sleep habits may ameliorate cardiovascular health. Metabolic Syndrome Metabolic pattern, a cluster of conditions including high blood pressure, insulin resistance, and abdominal rotundity, is associated with sleep disturbances and dysregulated blood sugar situations. 6. Strategies for perfecting Sleep and Blood Sugar Regulation To optimize the sleep- blood sugar connection and promote overall health, consider the following strategies Prioritize Sleep insure you get an acceptable quantum of sleep each night, generally between 7 to 9 hours for grown-ups. produce a sleep-friendly terrain and establish a harmonious sleep schedule. Ameliorate Sleep Quality Address any sleep disturbances or diseases, similar as sleep apnea or wakefulness. Exercise relaxation ways before bedtime to ameliorate sleep quality. Maintain a Healthy life Engage in regular physical exertion, eat a balanced diet, and manage stress situations, as these factors can appreciatively impact blood sugar regulation and sleep.   Limit Screen Time Before Bed Exposure to blue light from electronic bias can disrupt the   product of sleep- promoting hormones like melatonin. Limit screen time at least an hour before bedtime.   Seek Professional Help still, consult a healthcare professional to identify and address underpinning causes, If you're passing habitual sleep issues or blood sugar imbalances.   sleep- blood sugar connection is a complex and critical aspect of mortal health. Understanding the relationship between sleep and blood sugar regulation can empower individualities to make informed life choices to support optimal well-being and reduce the threat of metabolic diseases. By prioritizing healthy sleep habits and   espousing strategies to ameliorate sleep quality, individualities can appreciatively impact their blood sugar situations and overall health in the long run.

Strategies for Better Blood Sugar Control during Sleep

Maintaining stable blood sugar levels is crucial for overall health, especially for individuals living with diabetes. During sleep, the body undergoes several metabolic changes, and blood sugar control becomes even more challenging. Proper management of blood glucose during sleep is essential to prevent nocturnal hypoglycemia or hyperglycemia, which can lead to serious health complications. In this article, we will explore effective strategies to achieve better blood sugar control during sleep, enabling individuals with diabetes to rest peacefully and wake up with improved health and well-being.

Regular Monitoring:

Consistent monitoring of blood sugar levels is the foundation of successful diabetes management. During sleep, fluctuations in blood sugar levels can occur due to various factors like dinner choices, exercise patterns, and medication doses. To ensure better blood sugar control, individuals should check their blood sugar levels before going to bed and, if necessary, set alarms for periodic checks throughout the night. Continuous glucose monitoring (CGM) systems can be especially helpful during sleep, as they provide real-time data, alerting users to any fluctuations in blood glucose levels.

Balanced Evening Meals:

The composition of the evening meal can significantly impact blood sugar levels during sleep. Opt for a balanced dinner that includes a mix of complex carbohydrates, lean proteins, and healthy fats. Complex carbs release glucose more steadily, preventing rapid spikes in blood sugar. Avoiding high-glycemic index foods and sugary snacks close to bedtime can help maintain stable blood sugar levels throughout the night.

Time-Restricted Eating:

Implementing time-restricted eating, also known as intermittent fasting, may benefit blood sugar control during sleep. By consuming all meals and snacks within a specific time window during the day, the body can better manage blood sugar levels. However, individuals with diabetes should consult their healthcare provider before adopting any fasting regimen to ensure it aligns with their treatment plan.

Regular Physical Activity:

Engaging in regular physical activity can help improve insulin sensitivity and blood sugar regulation. Exercising earlier in the day rather than close to bedtime is recommended, as it gives the body ample time to recover and prevents any potential disruptions to sleep patterns. Moderate-intensity exercises such as walking, swimming, or cycling can be beneficial for managing blood sugar levels.

Medication and Insulin Management:

Proper medication and insulin management are vital for controlling blood sugar during sleep. Some diabetes medications may increase the risk of nocturnal hypoglycemia, while others might have a stronger effect during the night. Work closely with a healthcare provider to adjust medication dosages and insulin regimens based on individual needs and lifestyle factors.

Stress Reduction and Relaxation Techniques:

Stress can trigger hormonal responses that influence blood sugar levels, making it essential to manage stress levels before bedtime. Incorporate relaxation techniques such as meditation, deep breathing exercises, or yoga into the evening routine to promote better sleep and help stabilize blood sugar.

Bedroom Environment:

Creating a conducive sleep environment can positively impact blood sugar control. Ensure the bedroom is cool, dark, and free from distractions, as quality sleep is crucial for maintaining overall health and optimal blood sugar regulation.

Bedtime Snacks:
For individuals prone to nocturnal hypoglycemia, a small bedtime snack may help stabilize blood sugar levels during sleep. Opt for snacks that combine protein and healthy fats with slow-releasing carbohydrates, such as a handful of nuts with a slice of whole-grain bread.

Hydration:
Staying adequately hydrated is essential for blood sugar regulation. However, avoid excessive fluid intake right before bedtime to prevent disruptions due to frequent trips to the bathroom during the night.

Consistent Sleep Schedule:
Establishing a regular sleep schedule helps the body's internal clock regulate various physiological processes, including blood sugar control. Strive for consistent sleep and wake times, even on weekends, to support stable blood glucose levels.

Achieving better blood sugar control during sleep is a crucial aspect of diabetes management. By implementing these strategies, individuals can improve their overall well-being and reduce the risk of diabetes-related complications. Remember to work closely with healthcare providers to tailor these strategies to individual needs and create a personalized plan for optimal blood sugar regulation during sleep.

CHAPTER 8
Addressing Other Health Factors for Optimal Blood Sugar Content

Maintaining optimal blood sugar situations is pivotal for overall health and well- being. unbridled blood sugar can lead to colorful health complications, including type 2 diabetes, cardiovascular complaint, and rotundity. While diet and exercise are generally known as primary factors impacting blood sugar content, several other health factors play a significant part in its regulation. In this composition, we will explore the significance of addressing these fresh health factors to achieve optimal blood sugar situations and promote a healthier life. Stress operation habitual stress can have a profound impact on blood sugar regulation. When stressed, the body releases stress hormones like cortisol and adrenaline, driving the liver to release glucose into the bloodstream. This process is called the" fight- or- flight" response, designed to give quick energy during extremities. still, in moment's fast- paced world, habitual stress can lead to constantly elevated blood sugar situations. Addressing stress through relaxation ways similar as awareness, contemplation, yoga, or engaging in pursuits can help lower stress hormone situations and promote better blood sugar control. Sleep Quality and Duration Acceptable sleep is vital for maintaining balanced blood sugar situations. Poor sleep patterns, like irregular sleep schedules or sleep privation, can disrupt insulin perceptivity and lead to insulin resistance, a condition where the body's cells don't respond effectively to insulin. icing a harmonious sleep schedule, creating a comforting bedtime routine, and avoiding instigations before bedtime can contribute to bettered sleep quality, therefore appreciatively impacting blood sugar regulation. Physical exertion Regular physical exertion is a foundation of blood sugar operation. Exercise helps increase insulin perceptivity, allowing the body to use glucose more effectively. It also aids in weight operation, reducing the threat of rotundity- related blood sugar imbalances. Incorporating a blend of aerobic exercises(like walking, jogging, or swimming) and strength training into bone's routine can help optimize blood sugar situations and overall health. Gut Health and Probiotics The gut microbiome, composed of trillions of bacteria, plays a pivotal part in colorful aspects of health, including blood sugar regulation. Studies have shown that an imbalance in gut bacteria can contribute to insulin resistance and metabolic diseases. Consuming probiotic-rich foods or supplements can support a healthy gut microbiome and ameliorate blood sugar control. Foods like yogurt, kefir, sauerkraut, and kimchi are excellent sources of probiotics. Hydration Staying doused is essential for maintaining balanced blood sugar situations. Dehumidification can lead to elevated blood sugar, as the feathers work less efficiently to remove redundant glucose from the bloodstream. Drinking plenitude of water throughout the day can help help dehumidification and support optimal blood sugar regulation.   Nutrition Besides the well- known impact of carbohydrates on blood sugar situations, other salutary factors can   impact blood sugar regulation. For illustration, foods high in refined sugars and unhealthy fats can beget   rapid-fire harpoons in blood sugar situations.   A balanced diet rich in fiber, whole grains, spare proteins, healthy fats, and a variety of fruits and vegetables can promote stable blood sugar situations and overall health.   Medication Management For individualities with diabetes or other blood sugar- related conditions, clinging to specified specifics is pivotal for blood sugar control. Proper drug operation, along with life changes, can significantly impact blood sugar situations and   help complications.   Conclusion Optimal blood sugar content isn't solely determined by diet and exercise; colorful other health factors play an integral   part in its regulation. Addressing stress, maintaining quality sleep, engaging in physical exertion, supporting gut health, staying doused , and espousing a balanced diet are all essential   factors of a comprehensive approach to blood sugar operation. By fastening on these factors, individualities can achieve better blood sugar control, reduce the threat of habitual conditions, and ameliorate overall well- being, leading to a healthier and further fulfilling life. Always consult with a healthcare professional before making significant life changes or starting any new treatment.

The Importance of Regular Health Checkups

Maintaining good health is a vital aspect of leading a fulfilling and productive life. Regular health checks play a vital part in this pursuit by enabling individualities to cover and manage their well- being effectively. These routine examinations serve as preventative measures, allowing for the early discovery and treatment of implicit health issues. In this essay, we will claw into the significance of regular health checks and punctuate the colorful benefits they offer to individualities and society as a whole.   First and foremost, regular health checks promote early discovery of health problems. frequently, individualities may not witness conspicuous symptoms in the   original stages of certain   ails. By the time symptoms come apparent, the condition may have advanced, making it more   grueling to treat. Regular checks,   still, allow healthcare professionals to conduct thorough assessments, including blood tests, wireworks, and physical examinations. Through these evaluations, implicit health issues can be linked in their early stages, adding   the liability of successful treatment and better issues.   also, health checks enable the operation of habitual conditions. numerous   individualities live with habitual   ails   similar as diabetes, hypertension, and heart complaint, among others. These conditions bear ongoing monitoring and care to   help complications. Regular health   checks help healthcare providers assess the progress of habitual conditions, acclimate treatment plans, and offer necessary life advice. With proper operation, individualities with habitual ails can lead   healthier   lives   and   reduce   the   threat   of complications, hospitalizations, and disability. likewise, health checks play a pivotal part in preventative healthcare. Prevention is incontrovertibly better and further cost-effective than treatment. By relating threat factors and making life variations, individualities can help the onset of multitudinous health conditions. Routine checks give openings for healthcare professionals to educate cases about healthy habits, similar as regular exercise, balanced nutrition, and stress operation. Armed with this knowledge, individualities can make informed choices that appreciatively impact their health and well- being. In addition to individual benefits, regular health checks contribute to the overall enhancement of public health. When a significant portion of the population participates in routine wireworks, the early discovery and constraint of contagious conditions come more doable. For case, regular vaccinations and wireworks for contagious conditions can help help outbreaks and safeguard communities. likewise, individualities who are apprehensive of their health status are more likely to take necessary preventives to avoid spreading infections to others. piecemeal from physical health, regular health checks also support internal well- being. The stress of ultramodern life can take a risk on internal health, leading to conditions like anxiety and depression. During health checks, healthcare professionals can interrogate about an existent's emotional well- being and give support or referrals to internal health specialists, if necessary. Addressing internal health enterprises at an early stage can help their exacerbation and help individualities lead happier and further fulfilling lives. Regular health checks also foster a stronger croake - case relationship. When individualities see their healthcare providers regularly, a fellowship develops, which encourages open communication and trust. Cases are more likely to partake enterprises and symptoms actually, enabling healthcare providers to make accurate judgments and substantiated treatment plans. This cooperation between cases and healthcare professionals is essential for achieving optimal health issues. also, regular health checks can lead to cost savings in the long run. preventative care is generally less precious than treating advanced health conditions. Beforehand discovery and intervention can help the need for expensive medical procedures and hospitalizations. also, by managing habitual ails effectively, individualities can reduce healthcare charges associated with complications and exigency care. Regular health checks are of consummate significance for maintaining overall well- being and precluding the progression of health issues. These routine examinations grease early discovery, operation of habitual conditions, and creation of preventative healthcare. They contribute not only to individual health but also to the broader enhancement of public health. By prioritizing regular health checks, individualities can take charge of their health, enhance their quality of life, and reduce the burden on healthcare systems. Embracing preventative care is a visionary step towards a healthier and further prosperous future for   individualities and society as a whole.

Conclusion

In conclusion, Managing Glucose, Enhancing Life: A Step-by-Step Approach to Blood Sugar Mastery presents a comprehensive and empowering guide for individuals seeking to take control of their blood sugar levels and improve their overall well-being. Through a holistic and proactive approach, this book offers valuable insights, practical strategies, and the motivation needed to embrace a healthier lifestyle and unlock the full potential of life.

The journey to blood sugar mastery is not just about managing glucose levels; it is a path towards self-discovery and a deeper understanding of one's body and mind. By adopting the step-by-step approach outlined in this book, individuals can pave the way to a balanced and harmonious life.

The first and fundamental step on this journey is knowledge. Understanding how glucose functions in the body, its impact on health, and the potential risks of uncontrolled blood sugar is paramount. Armed with this knowledge, readers can make informed decisions about their diet, exercise routines, and overall lifestyle choices.

Through practical tips on nutrition, physical activity, and stress management, Managing Glucose, Enhancing Life enables readers to cultivate healthy habits that will not only stabilize blood sugar levels but also enhance their vitality and energy levels. By empowering individuals to make mindful food choices, engage in regular exercise, and develop effective stress-coping mechanisms, this book fosters a positive transformation that extends far beyond glucose management.

The significance of the mind-body connection cannot be understated. A positive and resilient mindset plays a pivotal role in blood sugar mastery. By promoting mindfulness, stress-reduction techniques, and fostering a sense of self-compassion, this book equips readers with powerful tools to confront life's challenges with newfound strength and determination.

Furthermore, Managing Glucose, Enhancing Life emphasizes the importance of community and support networks. Building a strong support system can make a world of difference for individuals striving to take control of their blood sugar. Whether it be through friends, family, or professional support groups, the journey to mastery becomes more manageable when shared with others.

As individuals progress on their blood sugar mastery journey, they may encounter setbacks or unforeseen challenges. This book acknowledges that setbacks are a natural part of any transformative process and provides guidance on how to rebound and maintain motivation. Embracing these challenges as learning opportunities and using them as stepping stones rather than stumbling blocks can lead to personal growth and long-term success.

Furthermore, Managing Glucose, Enhancing Life encourages readers to celebrate their victories, no matter how small. Each positive step taken towards blood sugar mastery is a cause for celebration and serves as a reminder of the progress made on the path to a healthier and more fulfilling life.

In a society increasingly affected by lifestyle-related health issues, the importance of blood sugar management cannot be underestimated. By taking charge of their blood sugar levels, individuals can potentially prevent or manage conditions like diabetes, reduce the risk of cardiovascular disease, and enhance overall longevity. As such, the impact of this book extends far beyond individual readers to positively influence the well-being of families, communities, and society as a whole.

Lastly, Managing Glucose, Enhancing Life: A Step-by-Step Approach to Blood Sugar Mastery serves as a beacon of hope and a roadmap for those seeking to reclaim their health and vitality. Through its comprehensive and empowering content, this book demonstrates that blood sugar mastery is not a mere medical necessity; it is a transformative journey towards enhanced life quality.

As readers implement the strategies and insights shared within these pages, they embark on a fulfilling and purpose-driven path to personal growth. By taking charge of their glucose levels, they are taking charge of their lives, enabling them to embrace each day with newfound energy, confidence, and joy.

So, whether you are a seasoned health enthusiast or someone who has just begun their quest for better health, Managing Glucose, Enhancing Life is a must-read. Together, let us embrace the principles outlined in this book and embark on a journey towards blood sugar mastery—a journey that promises to enhance not only our own lives but also the lives of those around us. Let us seize this opportunity to transform ourselves, our communities, and our world, one step at a time.